Country-Western
DANCING

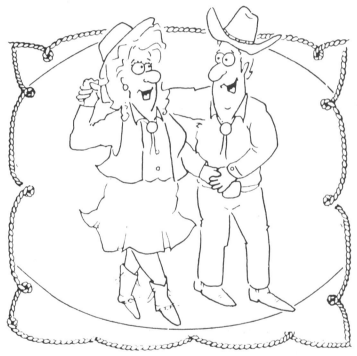

Barry Nelson

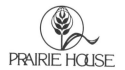

PRAIRIE HOUSE

Prairie House Inc.
P.O. Box 9199
Fargo, North Dakota 58106-9199

ISBN 0-911007-29-6

Illustration: © John Kolness 1993

Quantity discounts are available for dance instructors and other purchasers of copies in bulk. For information, write Prairie House, Inc., or call 1–800–866–BOOK (1–800–866–2665).

Special thanks to John Kolness for his art and advice, and to Terri Evans and other fine friends for teaching me how much fun dancing can be.

This book is dedicated to my parents, Nordal and Shirley, who not too long ago passed away ... they are greatly missed.

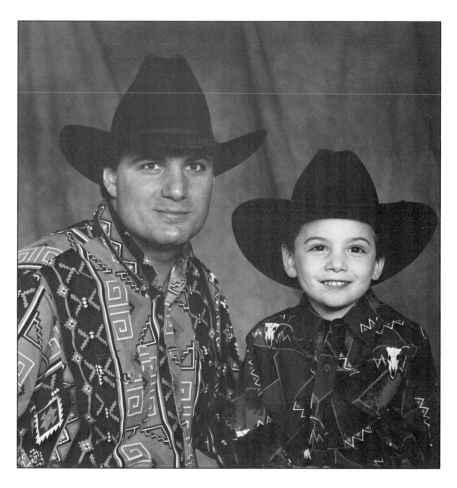

About the Author

Author Barry Nelson, a native of Hendrum, Minnesota, is one of the six children of Nordal and Shirley Nelson. A 1982 graduate of Hendrum-Perley High School, he attended the University of Minnesota Crookston and Moorhead Technical College. He has one son, his pride and joy, four-year-old Cody.

Barry started dancing in February 1992. Instantly he was hooked! Within weeks he was teaching country-western dancing throughout the Fargo, North Dakota–Moorhead, Minnesota, area. This handbook grew out of his experiences teaching hundreds and hundreds of country-western music fans to get up onto their feet and become a part of America's fastest growing dance scene.

Table of Contents

Welcome to the Excitement Of Country–Western Dancing

The ever–growing popularity of country music is matched only by enthusiasm for country-western dancing. The time has come for a step-by-step guide — a useful tool for those interested in learning the country-western dances.

I certainly can't take credit for creating the dances included in this handbook. Nor do I claim to be a so-called "dance expert." If you get the chance to take a class from one of the many good instructors across the country, do go ahead and take lessons. In the meantime, this book may give you a hand in getting started.

Country-western dancing is great family fun and a great way to enjoy your favorite music.

Good luck, have fun ... and thank you!

Barry Nelson

Dance–Floor Traffic Flow Pattern

☐ **More advanced dancers:** Stay toward the outside of the dance-floor flow.

☐ **Less advanced dancers:** Stay toward the inner portion of the dance-floor flow.

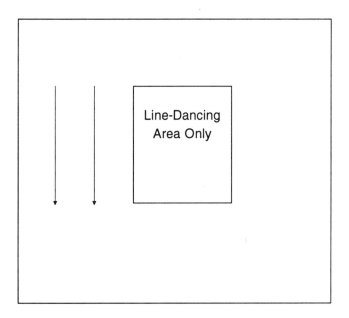

Dance–Floor Etiquette

Every dancer needs to follow a few simple rules to insure that everyone has a great time dancing:

- [ ] The dance–floor traffic flow pattern is a continuous, smooth-flowing pattern that moves in the counter-clockwise direction.
- [ ] Dancers with more experience who are moving at a quicker pace should stay toward the outer portion of the dance floor.
- [ ] Dancers with less experience moving at a slower pace should stay towards the inner portion of the dance floor.
- [ ] Dancers in the inner portion of the dance floor must be aware of line dancers, who are generally using the middle of the dance floor. Be conscious of them — don't squeeze their designated area.
- [ ] Line dancing is generally done in the middle of the dance floor, in an imaginary rectangular space, unless a particular club specifies another location.
- [ ] Traditional dancers must never cut across the line-dance area. This rule helps to avoid collisions and/or injuries.
- [ ] Line dancers must stay in their designated areas.
- [ ] As the floor fills with traditional dancers, line dancers need to be courteous. Take smaller steps so you do not take up unnecessary space on the dance floor.
- [ ] All dancers should be aware of everyone around them. Look around. Anticipate your neighbors' movements; maneuver in a way to avoid congestion and/or collisions.
- [ ] Collisions or minor bumping into other people *will* occur while you're dancing. When this happens, be polite and courteous regardless of who bumped whom.

NOTICE: Some of the dances detailed in this book may be somewhat different from the versions you are used to. There are lots of dances out there along with many variations!

Examples of appropriate music are noted at the end of each dance to suggest the rhythm that works best. Of course, no dance is limited to the songs I've suggested.

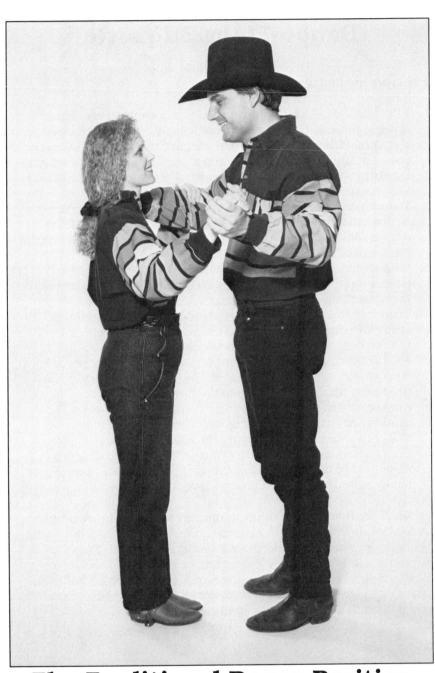

The Traditional Dance Position

Traditional Dance Position

The gentleman starts in the forward position in relation to the dance-floor traffic-flow pattern, facing his partner. The gentleman's right arm should be straight, with the elbow slightly bent for comfort. His right hand rests on the lady's left shoulder. (Men, remember not to have a heavy hand!)

Gentleman, keep the thumb of your right hand towards your index finger, and not in front of your partner's neck. Your right hand resting on your partner's left shoulder is known as the "gentlemen's controlling hand" or "lead." In this position, the gentleman should be able to lead his partner around on the dance floor, not by talking but by his signals.

Here are some examples of signals:

When the gentleman wishes to start moving forward in the dance floor traffic flow pattern, he gently pushes forward with the heel of his right hand against the front of his partner's left shoulder. This is the lady's signal to begin her dance steps going backward in relation to the traffic-flow pattern.

If the dance traffic ahead is heavy and congested, the gentleman applies pressure with the fingertips of his right hand against the back of the lady's left shoulder. Men, by using this signal, you are halting your partner from moving backward in her line of dance; yet you both continue to dance — but in place. When congestion ahead clears enough to continue in your line of dance, the gentleman releases his finger pressure and gently pushes forward with the heel of his right hand, signaling his partner to continue moving.

The man should also be able to signal his partner of directional changes by moving his wrist from side to side, with just enough pressure to signal to his partner what his intentions are and what he expects from her.

Ladies, when you are going forward in the traffic-flow pattern and the gentleman is going backward, you too must watch traffic ahead. If traffic gets heavy or congested, you gently squeeze the gentleman's right arm with your left hand; this signals him to halt and dance in place. Release the squeeze pressure to signal that the congestion ahead has eased.

In the traditional dance position — with the gentleman's controlling hand in position — the lady's left hand should gently rest over the gentleman's arm between his elbow and shoulder. (Remember, ladies, not to have a heavy hand). Gentlemen, your left arm should be extended outward to your left side with a slightly bent elbow. The exact position will depend on your partner's height and what is comfortable for both of you.

The lady's right hand will rest between the man's thumb and index finger; neither partner should grip the other's hand. The proper hold or position is called a pressure hold. For example, imagine that you and your partner are holding a plate of glass between your hands, holding it in place only by the pressure being applied by the palms of your hands. (When you and your partner start getting into turns, spins and so on, you'll realize it's much easier if your hands aren't gripped tightly together).

This is the traditional dance position. When you begin, you step at the same time. The gentleman starts with his left foot first, and the lady with her right foot first. This applies whether you're starting forward or backward in the dance-floor traffic-flow pattern.

The Texas Two-Step (Basic Steps)

The basic pattern is Long, Long, Short-Short.....or.....Slow, Slow, Quick-Quick.

Gentlemen's steps are: Left, Right, Left-Right (REPEATING).

NOTE: *The first two steps (Long) are taken with normal strides, and the next two steps (Short) are about one-half the span of the (Long) strides.*

The basic steps are the same for the ladies — Long, Long, Short-Short — but their leads are exactly opposite. The man's first stride is taken with his left foot first; so, ladies, your first stride will be taken with your right foot.

Ladies, your steps are: Right, Left, Right-Left (REPEATING).

The Texas Two-Step steps are progressive steps forward or backward, not from side to side, not swaying your torso or hips, and definitely not rapidly pumping your arms up and down. By dancing smoothly and gracefully, both partners appear to be more beautiful and elegant.

The Three-Step (Basic Steps)

First, let's say that the music is either too fast or too slow for the Texas Two-Step, and isn't a waltz beat. What do you do? In order to move with the beats of the music, you may want to do the Three-Step (Shuffle Steps). The art of recognizing the up and down beats of the music comes naturally for some, but may take some folks a little longer. Identifying the beats of the music is a key element in deciding what type of dance you and your partner should do.

In the Three-Step, the steps are shorter and quicker — like shuffle steps, either forward or backward. The step count is: 1&2 ... 3&4 ... 1&2 ... 3&4.

Gentlemen: The steps are Left, Right, Left ... Right, Left, Right ... Left, Right, Left ... Right, Left, Right (and so on). The steps keep repeating. Note that on the (1) and the (3) you will be leading with alternating steps.

Ladies: Your count is the same — 1&2 ... 3&4 and so on. But your steps (as in the Texas Two-Step) are the mirror image of the gentleman's steps. You will start with your right foot.

The Waltz (Basic Steps)

I believe the waltz is the most elegant dance, especially if done correctly by a couple dancing with strict form.

The step count to the waltz is: 1-2-3 ... 4-5-6 ... 1-2-3 ... 4-5-6 (repeating). Or you may count your steps as Long-Short-Short ... Long-Short-Short.

Note that on the (1) and (4) counts you will alternate your lead steps: Left—Right—Left ... Right—Left—Right (repeating).

Gentlemen, this is the waltz:

1-Step forward with your left foot.

2-Bring your right foot to your left foot.

3-Step in place with your left foot alongside your right foot.

4-Step forward with your right foot.

5-Bring your left foot to your right foot.

6-Step in place with your right foot alongside your left foot.

REPEAT THIS SEQUENCE

Ladies, once again your step count is the same as the gentleman's and the strides are with the same approximate span. However, ladies, your steps are the mirror image of your male counterpart. Start with your right foot.

Examples of Waltz music..

□ *You Look So Good in Love*.....George Strait.

□ *Here's a Quarter*.....Travis Tritt.

□ *New Way to Fly*.....Garth Brooks.

□ *Walkin' Away*.....Clint Black.

□ *Could I Have This Dance*.....Ann Murray.

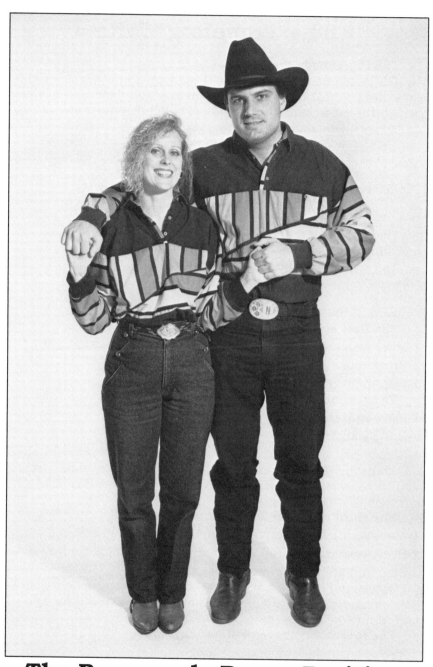

The Promenade Dance Position

The Traveling Waltz

The Promenade Position:

The gentleman stands beside the lady, with both facing the same direction. The gentleman's right arm goes behind the lady's neck, with the weight of his arm resting lightly on her shoulders.

The gentleman cups the lady's left hand in his right hand. The gentleman's left arm is bent at a 90° angle and held directly in front and across his stomach, with the hand cupped with hers.

Both start with your left foot.

Remember, the waltz steps are: Long-Short-Short ... Long-Short-Short alternating you lead foot every series of Long-Short-Shorts.

The pattern of the dance has 10 sequences which keep repeating as the dance continues.

The pattern of the dance:

Forward ... Back ... Right side ...
Left side ... Right side ... Left side ...
Forward ... Back ... Forward ... Back.

The first sequence of steps: *Forward.*

1-Move your left foot forward=(long).

2-Bring your right foot to your left foot=(short).

3-Step in place with your left foot=(short).

The second sequence of steps: *Back.*

4-Move your right foot back=(long).

5-Bring your left foot to your right foot=(short).

6-Step in place with your right foot=(short).

Now after doing a quarter-turn to your right using your last two short-short steps, you should now be facing a different direction.

The third sequence of steps: *Right side.*

1-Move your left foot forward=(long).

2-Bring your right foot to your left=(short).

3-Step in place with your left foot=(short).

As you did sequence No. 3, on the last two steps (short-shorts) you should have been stepping in a manner as to complete a half-turn to the left.

The fourth sequence of steps: *Left side.*

4-Move your right foot forward=(long).

5-Bring your left foot to your right foot=(short).

6-Step in place with your right foot=(short).

Again, as did your last two short-short steps you should have been stepping in a manner as to complete a half-turn to the right.

(Confused yet? Refer to the "pattern of the dance" on the preceding page.)

The fifth sequence of steps: *Right side.*

1-Move your left foot forward=(long).

2-Bring your right foot to your left foot=(short).

3-Step in place with your left foot=(short).

Again, as you did your last two short-short steps you should have been stepping in a manner as to complete a half-turn to the left.

The sixth sequence of steps: *Left side.*

4-Move your right foot forward=(long).

5-Bring your left foot to your right foot=(short).

6-Step in place with your right foot=(short).

This time, as you did your last two short-short steps you should have been stepping in a manner as to complete a quarter-turn to the right.

The seventh sequence of steps: *Forward.*

1-Move your left foot forward=(long).

2-Bring your right foot to your left foot=(short).

3-Step in place with your left foot=(short).

The eighth sequence of steps: *Back.*

4-Move your right foot back=(long).

5-Bring your left foot to your right foot=(short).

6-Step in place with your right foot=(short).

The ninth sequence of steps: *Forward.*

1-Take your first step (long) with your left foot and turn a quarter-turn to the left at the same time. Gentlemen, raise your right hand (still holding hers) over her head.

By completing this quarter-turn, you are facing the left side and, ladies, you are directly facing your partner's back.

2-At this stage, disconnect your right hands while stepping down on your right foot (short).

3-At the same time, gentlemen, begin to raise your left hand (still holding hers) over her head while stepping a quarter-pivot turn back with your left foot (short).

At this point, you should join right hands again in front and you have now reversed your direction.

4-Now step back with your right foot=(long).

5-Bring your left foot to your right foot=(short).

6-Step in place with your right foot=(short).

The tenth sequence of steps: *Back.*

1-Step quarter-pivot turn to the left (long) while still holding
    hands.

*Now ladies are facing their left, and men are directly facing the
ladies' backs.*

2-Step quarter-pivot turn back with your right foot (short).

NOTE: *While stepping this step, bring your left hands down,
still connected, and raise your right hands into the promenade
position.*

3-Step in place with your left foot=(short).

*At this point you will be facing the front again as you were
when you started this dance.*

4-Step back with your right foot=(long).

5-Bring your left foot to your right foot=(short).

6-Step in place with your right foot=(short).

   REPEAT ALL SEQUENCES

Music for Traveling Waltz
☐   *You Look So Good In Love*.....George Strait.
☐   *New Way To Fly*.....Garth Brooks.

The Traveling Four Corners

This a couples dance, done in a circular pattern around the dance floor. The gentleman's right arm will extend across the back of his partner's shoulders holding her right hand in his. The gentleman's left arm will be bent at a 90° angle against his stomach, cupping her left hand in his. Yes, you're side by side, and will begin facing into the inner portion of the dance floor.

1,2-Move your left leg forward and tap your heel to the floor in front of your right foot and return.

3,4-Move your right leg forward and tap your heel to the floor in front of your left foot and return.

1-Step out to your left side with your left foot.

2-Step behind your left foot with your right foot.

3-Step out to your left side with your left foot.

4-Brush forward with your right foot.

1-Step out to your right side with your right foot.

2-Step behind your right foot with your left foot.

3-Step out to your right side with your right foot pointing your toes to the far right.

4-Brush with your left foot and complete the half-turn to your right.

1-Step to your left side with your left foot.

2-Step behind your left foot with your right foot.

3-Step out to your left with your left foot pointing your toes to the far left.

4-Brush with your right foot and complete the half-turn to your left and stepping down on your right foot.
REPEAT

Music for Traveling Four Corners Line Dance
☐ *Ain't Nothin' Wrong With the Radio*.....Aaron Tippin.
☐ *Whiskey Ain't Workin'*.....Travis Tritt.

The Traveling Cha–Cha

Start with the gentleman's right arm behind his lady partner's neck and resting across the back of her shoulders holding her right hand in his. Gentlemen, your left arm will be bent at 90° and *behind* your back with your forearm pressed against your back with your left hand cupped to cup her left hand.

NOTE: *When doing the half-turns your hands stay connected most of the time, to complete the turns with your hands connected you'll be using over–the–head windmill–type movements with your arms. I think trying to explain this dance with words is much harder than the actual dance, but we'll give it a try. This dance does not travel around the dance floor, so do this dance in the line dance area, as long as there isn't a line dance being done.*

3-Rock forward on your left foot.

4-Rock back on your right foot.

1,2,3-Move backward with small and quick (Cha, Cha, Cha) steps: left, right, left.

4-Rock back on your right foot.

1-Move your right foot forward, point your toes to your far left...(Cha).

2-Move your left foot back, completing a quarter-turn to your left...(Cha).

3-Move your right foot back, completing a quarter-turn to your left...(Cha).

4-Rock back on your left foot.

1-Moving your left foot forward, point your toes to your far right...(Cha) .

2-Move your right foot back, completing a quarter-turn to your right...(Cha).

3-Move your left foot back, completing another quarter-turn to your left...(Cha).

4-Rock back on your right foot.

1,2,3,4-MEN-Move your right foot forward and do a right, left, right (Cha-Cha-Cha) in place then do a rock step out to your left side. While you are doing this, with your first (Cha) step you let go of her left hand and at the same time raise your right arm up and lead your partner into a counter-clockwise (Cha-Cha-Cha) half-spinning turn.

1,2,3,4-WOMEN-At the same exact time the man is doing his (Cha-Cha-Cha) steps in place, you will move your right foot first and turn counter-clockwise as you do your (Cha-Cha-Cha) steps: right, left, right—then, stepping slightly back with your left foot, do a rock step.

At this point, ladies, you will do the mirror image of your partners' moves.

1-M/W-Step towards your right with your left foot (quarter-turn).

2-M/W-From this position, do a half-turn pivot on the balls of your feet to the right. The gentleman will pass under his arm while he pivots then raising it first from in front of his face to over the back of his partner's head. You have completed a half-turn and are now in position to join hands together again behind his back.

Gentlemen, note that you leave your left hand in position behind your back whether you're holding her left hand or not.

REPEAT

Music for Traveling Cha-Cha

☐ *Neon Moon*.....Brooks & Dunn.

☐ *If I Could Bottle This Up*.....Paul Overstreet.

The Sierra Rose

This dance is done in a circle in a guy-girl alternating pattern. In the first four segments of this dance the men and women will move simultaneously and yet be doing slightly different steps.

1,2-M-Step forward with your right foot and pivot half-turn to the left.

1,2-W-Fan the toes of your right foot to the right and return to normal stance.

3,4-M-Step forward with your right foot and pivot half-turn to the left.

3,4-W-Fan the toes of your right foot to the right and return to normal stance.

1,2-M-Move your right foot forward and tap your heel to the floor and return.

1,2-W-Step forward with your right foot and pivot half-turn to the left.

3,4-M-Move your right foot forward and tap your heel to the floor and return.

3,4-W-Step forward with your right foot and pivot half-turn to the left.

Now both men and women:

1-Step forward with your right foot.

2-Step forward bringing your left foot alongside your right foot.

3,4-Kick downward and forward, twice (into the circle) with your right foot.

1-Step back with your right foot.

2-Move backward with your left foot touching your toes to the floor.

3-Step forward with your left foot.

4-Step forward bringing your right foot alongside your left foot.

1,2-Kick downward and forward, twice, with your left foot.

3-Step out to your left side with your left foot.

4-Step behind your left foot with your right foot.

1-Step out to the left side with your left foot.

2-Slide your right foot together with your left foot and clap your hands.

3-Step out to the right side with your right foot.

4-Slide your left foot together with your right foot and clap your hands.

1-Step out to the left side with your left foot.

2-Slide your right foot together with your left foot and clap your hands.

3-Step out to your right side with your right foot.

4-Step behind your right foot with your left foot.

1-Step out to your right side with your right foot pointing your toes to the far right.

2-Do a half-turn to your right with a brush of your left foot against the floor.

3-Step to your left side with your left foot.

4-Step behind your left foot with your right foot.

1-Step out to your left side with your left foot.

2-Do a half-turn to your left with a brush of your right foot against the floor.

3,4-Stomp in place with your right foot, twice.

REPEAT

Music for Sierra Rose

☐ *Except For Monday*.....Lorrie Morgan.

☐ *Mirror, Mirror*.....Diamond Rio.

The Wooden Nickel

This dance is done with the gentleman standing beside his lady partner in the promenade position. The dance will travel around the dance floor in a counter-clockwise direction.

1-Step forward with your left foot.

2-Step forward with your right foot.

3-Step forward with your left foot.

4,1,2-Scuff the floor in a forward motion with your right foot and kick with a downward motion like you are applying the breaks of your car, twice.

3-Step down and forward with your right foot.

4-Step forward with your left foot.

1-Step forward with your right foot.

2,3,4-Scuff the floor in a forward motion with your left foot and kick with a downward motion like you are applying the breaks of your car, twice.

1-Step down and forward with your left foot.

2-Bring your right foot to your left foot.

3-Step a quarter-turn to your left with your left foot.

   NOTE: *At this point the gentleman will be facing the inner portion of the dance floor with his lady partner directly behind him, facing his back. The gentleman's right arm will be bent up at 90˚, and his right hand will be bent back at 90˚ with your palms up. The lady's right hand will rest palms down on the gentleman's hand as for now your left hand will rest on your own left hip.*

4-Bring your right foot alongside your left foot.

1-Step out to your right side with your right foot.

&-Step behind your right foot with your left foot.

2-Step out to your right side with your right foot.

&-Step behind your right foot with your left foot.

3-Step out to your right side with your right foot.

&-Step behind your right foot with your left foot.

4-Step out to your right side with your right foot, pointing your toes to the far right.

&-Brush the floor as you swing your left leg around completing a half-turn to the right.

1-And in the same motion, step with your left foot out to your left side.

NOTE: *While doing the half-turn, your right hands do not disconnect; but as you turn, raise them and rotate your palms. Now gentlemen should be facing the outside of the dance floor with your partners directly in front of you.*

&-Step behind your left foot with your right foot.

2-Step out to your left side with your left foot.

&-Step behind your left foot with your right foot.

3-Step out to your left side with your left foot.

&-Step behind your left foot with your right foot.

4-Step out to your left side with your left foot pointing your toes to the far left.

&-Brush the floor as you swing your right leg around.

1-Step down in place on your right foot turning one-third-turn to the left.

&-Scuff the floor in place with your left foot.
   NOTE: *You'll continue to circle.*

2-Step down with your left foot, in place, pointing your toes one-third-turn to the left.

&-Scuff the floor in place with your right foot (NOTE: You'll continue to circle.)

3-Step down in place with your right foot turning one-third-turn to the left.

&,4-Scuff in place with a forward motion with your left foot then step down on it.
   NOTE: *You have just completed a 360° turn, and while doing so your hands should have stayed connected, rotating upon each other's hand. Your shoulders at this point should be just as you started this dance, right shoulders toward the outside of the dance floor in promenade position.*

1&2-(Stepping down) do shuffle steps forward—left-right-left.

3&4-Do shuffle steps forward—right-left-right.
                    REPEAT

Music for Wooden Nickel
☐   *Two Of A Kind*.....Garth Brooks.
☐   *Boot Scootin' Boogie*.....Brooks & Dunn.

The Continental Cowboy

This is a partners dance. Ladies, you will be at the gentlemen's right side and will hold his right hand with your left.

1-M-Step out to your left side with your left foot.

1-W-Step out to your right side with your right foot.

2-M-Step behind your left foot with your right foot.

2.W-Step behind your right foot with your left foot.

3-M-Step out to your left side with your left foot.

3-W-Step out to your right side with your right foot.

4-M-Kick with your right foot angling it to the left.

4-W-Kick with your left foot angling it to the right.

1-M-Step to your right side with your right foot.

1-W-Step to your left side with your left foot.

2-M-Step behind your right foot with your left foot.

2-W-Step behind your left foot with your right foot.

3-M-Step to your right side with your right foot.

3-W-Step to your left side with your left foot.

4-M-Moving your left leg in front of you and up about 4-6", bump the inside of your left foot against the inside of your partner's right foot.

4-W-Moving your right leg in front of you and up about 4-6", bump the inside of your right foot against the inside of your partner's left foot.

1-M-Move your left foot out to the left side and touch the ball of your foot to the floor.

1-W-Move your right foot out to the right side and touch the ball of your foot the floor.

2-M-Moving your left leg behind your right calf, bump the inside of your left foot against the inside of your partner's right foot.

2-W-Moving your right leg behind your left calf, bump the inside of your right foot against the inside of your partner's left foot.

3-M-Move your left foot out to your left side and touch the floor.

3-W-Move your right foot out to your right side and touch the floor.

4-M-Bring your left foot back alongside your right foot.

4-W-Bring your right foot back alongside your left foot.

1,2-M-Do a heel swish to the left and return to normal stance.

1,2-W-Do a heel swish to the left and return to normal stance.

3,4-M-Do a heel swish to the right and return to normal stance.

3,4-W-Do a heel swish to the right and return to normal stance.

THEN DO SHUFFLE STEPS FORWARD:

1&2-M-Right, Left, Right.

1&2-W-Left, Right, Left.

3&4-M-Left, Right, Left.

3&4-W-Right, Left, Right.

1&2-M-Right, Left, Right.

1&2-W-Left, Right, Left.

REPEAT, TRAVELING COUNTER-CLOCKWISE AROUND THE DANCE FLOOR

Music for Continental Cowboy
- *Two Of A Kind*.....Garth Brooks.
- *Some Folks Like To Steal*.....Kentucky Head Hunters.

The Montana

This line dance is done with the gentlemen in a side-by-side line with about an arm's length between them. The ladies will form another side-by-side line facing their partners.

1,2-Pigeon toe.

3,4-Pigeon toe.

1-Move your right foot forward and touch your heel to the floor.

2-Bring your right foot back to your normal stance.

3-Move your right foot forward and touch your heel to the floor.

4-Bring your right foot back to your normal stance.

1,2-Pigeon toe.

3,4-Pigeon toe.

1-Move your left foot forward and touch your heel to the floor.

2-Bring your left foot back to your normal stance.

3-Move your left foot forward and touch your heel to the floor.

4-Bring your left foot back and touch your toes to the floor.

1-Step forward with your left foot.

2-Hitch up and forward with your right knee and do a "paddy-cake" clap with your partner.

3-Step back with your right foot.

4-Stomp your left foot alongside your right foot.

1-Step out to the left with your left foot.

2-Step behind your left foot with your right foot.

3-Step out to the left with your left foot.

4-Brush the floor with your right foot alongside your left foot.

1-Step out to the right with your right foot.

2-Step behind your right foot with your left foot.

3-Step quarter-turn to the right with your right foot.

4-Brush the floor with your left foot alongside your right foot.

1-Step out to the left with your left foot.

   NOTE: *Ladies' and gentlemen's lines will cross each other.*

2-Step behind your left foot with your right foot.

3-Step quarter-turn to the left with your left foot.

4-Swing your right leg one-third-turn to the left while brushing the floor with your right foot and pivoting to the left on your left foot.

1-Step down with your right foot.

2-Step down with your left foot.

NOTE: *Ladies' and gentlemen's lines will again be facing each other.*

3-Stomp (In place) with your right foot.

4-Stomp (In place) with your left foot.

REPEAT

Music for The Montana
☐ *Country Club*.....Travis Tritt.
☐ *Stand Up*.....Mel McDaniel.

The Schottische

1-Step out to the left with your left foot.

2-Step behind your left foot with your right foot.

3-Step out to the left with your left foot.

4-Hitch up with your right knee.

1-Step down and to the right with your right foot.

2-Step behind your right foot with your left foot.

3-Step out to the right with your right foot.

4-Hitch up with your left knee.

1-Step down and forward on your left foot.

2-Hitch up with your right knee.

3-Step down and forward on your right foot.

4-Hitch up with your left knee.

1-Step down and forward on your left foot.

2-Hitch up with your right knee.

3-Step down and forward on your right foot.

4-Hitch up with your left knee.

REPEAT

Note: *The Schottische is done as a couple, with gentleman's right arm extended across the shoulders of his partner holding her right hand. The gentleman's left arm will be at a 90 degree angle pressed against his stomach cupping his hand with her left hand. Yes, you are side by side, with the gentleman on the lady's left.*

This dance is done in a circular pattern going around the dance floor, going in the same direction as the normal traffic flow pattern.

Music for the Schottische
☐ *Schottische*.....Isaac Payton Sweat.

The Cherokee Kick

This dance is done in a circle with a gentleman-lady alternating pattern and the dancers facing into the circle.

1,2-On the balls of your feet, swish your heels to the right, then back to normal position.

3,4-Move your right foot forward and touch your heel to the floor and return.

1-Step forward with your right foot.

2-Kick forward with your left foot.

3-Bring your left foot back.

4-Bring your right foot back and touch your toes to the floor.

1-Step forward with your right foot.

2-Kick forward with your left foot.

3-Step back with your left foot.

4-Bring your right foot alongside your left foot.

1-Step to the right with your right foot.

2-Slide your left foot to your right foot. (Clap Hands).

3-Step to the left with your left foot.

4-Slide your right foot to your left foot (Clap Hands).

1-Step to the right with your right foot.

2-Step behind your right foot with your left foot.

3-Step one-third-turn to the right with your right foot.

4-Hitch up with your left knee bent while pivoting one-third-turn to the right.

1-Step down with your left foot with one-third-turn to the right.

2-Hitch up with your right knee while pivoting one-third-turn to the right.

3-Step down on your right foot with one-third-turn to the right.

4-Hitch up with your left knee.

At this point, all dancers should still be in their circle with the right side of their bodies toward the outside of the circle.

1-Step down and forward with your left foot.

2-Step forward with your right foot.

3,4-Hitch up with your left knee bent and hop forward, twice.

1-Step down and forward with your left foot.

2-Step forward with your right foot.

3-Step forward with your left foot doing quarter-turn to the left.

4-Stomp your right foot alongside your left foot.

Dancers should now be facing into the circle again.
REPEAT

Music for the Cherokee Kick
- ☐ *Lovin' all Night*.....Rodney Crowell.
- ☐ *Hold on Partner*.....Clint Black/Roy Rogers.

The Cotton-Eyed Joe

This dance starts with couples in the promenade position; they will travel around the dance floor in a counter-clockwise direction.

- Move your left foot to cross over in front of your right foot then kick forward with your left foot.
- Now do shuffle steps backward Left, Right, Left.
- Move your right foot to cross over in front of your left foot then kick forward with your right foot.
- Now do shuffle steps backward Right, Left, Right.
- Move your left foot to cross over in front of your right foot then kick forward with your left foot.
- Now do shuffle steps backward Left, Right, Left.
- Move your right foot to cross over in front of your left foot then kick forward with your right foot.
- Now do shuffle steps backward Right, Left, Right.

The Cotton-Eyed Joe continues by moving forward in a 3-step pattern, or shuffle steps, for 8 counts.

- Left, Right, Left (1&2).
- Right, Left, Right (3&4).
- Left, Right, Left (1&2).
- Right, Left, Right (3&4).
- Left, Right, Left (1&2).
- Right, Left, Right (3&4).
- Left, Right, Left (1&2).
- Right, Left, Right (3&4).

REPEAT

Music for the Cotton-Eyed Joe
- ☐ *Cotton-Eyed Joe*.....Isaac Payton Sweat.

The Southside Shuffle

This dance is done with a guy-girl alternating pattern, or with men in one line about an arm's length apart facing their lady partners in another line.

1,2-With your right foot (Fan) or swish your toes out to the right and return to normal stance.

3,4-Again, fan your right foot and return to normal stance.

1,2-Move your right leg forward and tap your right heel to the floor, twice.

3,4-Move your right leg backward and tap your toes to the floor twice.

1,2-Move your right leg forward, tap your heel to the floor and return to normal stance.

3-Move your right leg out to your right side, touching the ball of your right foot to the floor.

4-Bring your right foot up and behind your left knee, and slap the heel of your right foot with your left hand.

1-Bring your right foot down, stepping out to your right side.

2-Step behind your right foot with your left foot.

3-Step out to your right side with your right foot.

4-Brush the floor with your left foot passing beside your right foot.

1-Step out to your left side with your left foot.

2-Step behind your left foot with your right foot.

3-Step and point your left foot to the left in a quarter-directional turn to the left.

4-Brush the floor with your right foot, and in same motion...

1-...step out to the right side with your right foot.

2-Step behind your right foot with your left foot.

3-Step out to your right side with your right foot pointing your toes to the far right.

4-Swing your left leg around clockwise brushing the floor and completing a quarter-turn.

, **NOTE:** *At this point you should be facing your partner but facing a different direction from which your started.*

1-Stomp in place with your left foot.

2-Stomp in place with your right foot.

3-Stomp in place with your left foot.

4-Stomp in place with your right foot.

REPEAT

□   *Except For Monday.....*Lorrie Morgan.
□   *Country Club.....*Travis Tritt.

The County Line Grind

This dance is done with the gentleman standing on his lady's left side in the promenade position. This dance will travel around the dance floor in a counter-clockwise direction.

1-Move your right leg forward and touch your heel to the floor.

2-Move your right leg to cross over in front of your left leg (touching toes only).

1&2-Moving your right leg forward, do shuffle steps: right, left, right.

1-Move your left leg forward and as you step down, rock forward on your left foot.

2-Rock back on your right foot.

1&2-Moving your left leg back do shuffle steps: left, right, left.

1-Stepping back with your right leg, rock back on your right foot.

2-Rock forward on your left foot.

1&2-Move your right leg forward and do shuffle steps: right, left, right.

1,2-Step forward with your left foot and do a half-turn pivot to your right.

1&2-Move your left leg forward doing shuffle steps: left, right, left.

1-Stepping forward with your right foot, do a quarter-turn to your left.

NOTE: *At this point the lady will be facing the outside of the dance floor with her partner still holding hands, directly behind her ... close.*

2—3,4-With your momentum carrying you into a knees bent forward stance: Rotate your hips to the right side — slowly, with knees bent, grind downward and bring your hip up to the left (using "sexy" body language) and repeat.

After coming up from your second GRIND, move with your right foot a quarter-turn to your left.

1&2-Shuffle step forward: right, left, right.

3&4-Shuffle step forward: left, right, left.

                        REPEAT

Music for County Line Grind
□   *Friends In Low Places.....*Garth Brooks.
□   *Neon Moon.....*Brooks & Dunn.

The Ten–Step

This dance, like the Sixteen Step, begins with couples in promenade position and will travel around the dance floor counter-clockwise.

1,2-Move your left heel forward and touch the floor and return.

3,4-Move your right leg back and touch your toes to the floor and return.

5-Move your right heel forward and touch the floor.

6-With your right leg, cross over in front of your left leg touching only toes to the floor.

7,8-Move your right heel forward and touch the floor and return to normal stance.

9-Move your left leg forward and touch your heel to the floor.

10-With your left leg, cross over in front of your right leg touching only your toes to the floor.

1&2-Shuffle steps forward: left, right, left.

3&4-Shuffle steps: right, left, right.

1&2-Shuffle steps: left, right, left.

3&4-Shuffle steps: right, left, right.

1&2-Shuffle steps: left, right, left.

3&4-Shuffle steps: right, left, right.

1&2-Shuffle steps: left, right, left.

3&4-Shuffle steps: right, left, right.

REPEAT

Music for Ten–Step
☐ *Neon Moon*.....Brooks & Dunn.
☐ *Two Of A Kind*.....Garth Brooks.

The Sixteen–Step

This dance is done as a couples dance in the promenade position. When doing the half-turns or military turns, you can do underarm or windmill turns or just drop hands.

1,2-Move your right leg forward and tap your heel to the floor and return to normal stance.

3,4-Move your right leg forward and tap your heel to the floor and return to normal stance.

5,6-Move your left leg forward and tap your heel to the floor and return to normal stance.

7,8-Move your right leg back and tap your toes to the floor and return to normal stance.

9,10-Move your left leg forward and tap your heel to the floor and return to normal stance.

11,12-Stomp in place with your right foot, twice.

13-Step forward with your right foot (arm/hand options, see above description).

14-Do a half-turn to your left.

15-Step forward with your right foot.

16-Do a half-turn to your left.

3&4-Shuffle steps: right, left, right.

1&2-Shuffle steps: left, right, left.

3&4-Shuffle steps: right, left, right.

1&2-Shuffle steps: left, right, left.
                    REPEAT

Music for Sixteen Step
☐   *Neon Moon*.....Brooks & Dunn.
☐   *Two Of A Kind*.....Garth Brooks

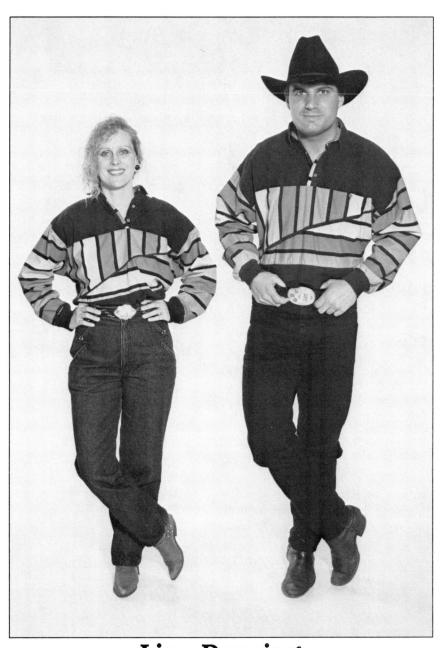

Line Dancing

The Hillbilly Cajun Slap Line Dance

Choreographed by Barry and Jerry Nelson

1-Step out to your right side with your right foot.

2-Step behind your right foot with your left foot.

3-Step out to your right side with your right foot.

4-Stomp your left foot alongside your right foot.

1-Move your left foot out to your left side.

2-Return your left foot alongside your right foot.

3-Move your left foot out to your left side.

4-Return your left foot alongside your right foot.

1-Step out to your left side with your left foot.

2-Step behind your left foot with your right foot.

3-Step out to your left side with your left foot.

4-Stomp your right foot alongside your left foot.

1-Move your right foot out to your right side.

2-Return your right foot alongside your left foot.

3-Move your right foot out to your right side.

4-Return your right foot alongside your left foot.

1,2-Move your right leg forward and tap your heel to the floor, twice.

3,4-Move your right leg back and tap your toes to the floor, twice.

1-Move your right leg forward and touch your right heel to the floor.

2-Raise your right leg up in hitch position and slap(with open hand/palms down)your right hand to the lower portion of your thigh.

3-Move your right leg so as to touch your right heel to the floor.

4-Bring your right leg up and slap the inside of your right heel with your open left hand.

1-Stepping down and forward with your right foot.

2-Do a half-turn pivot to your left.

3-Move your right leg forward and tap your heel to the floor.

4-Bring your right leg back beside your left leg.

REPEAT

Music for Hillbilly Cajun Slap Line Dance.

☐ *Country Club*.....Travis Tritt.

☐ *Ridin' The Rodeo*.....Vince Gill.

The Cowboy Stomp
(Honky–Tonk Stomp)

1,2-Pigeon toe.

3,4-Pigeon toe.

1-Move your right foot forward and touch your heel to the floor.

2-Bring your right foot back to your normal stance.

3-Move your right foot forward and touch your heel to the floor.

4-Bring your right foot back to your normal stance.

1,2-Stomp in place, twice, with your left foot.

3-Move your left foot forward and touch your heel to the floor.

4-Bring your left foot back to your normal stance.

1,2-Stomp in place, twice, with your right foot.(pause)

1-Step out to the right side with your right foot.

2-Step behind your right foot with your left foot.

3-Step out to the right with your right foot.

4-Brush with your left foot alongside your right foot.

1-Step out to the left side with your left foot.

2-Step behind your left foot with your right foot.

3-Step to the left with your left foot, pointing your toes to the far left.

4-Swing your right leg around your left leg, completing a half-turn to the left.

    NOTE: *At this point you should be facing the opposite of the direction in which you started.*

1-Step out to the right with your right foot.

2-Step behind your right foot with your left foot.

3-Step out to the right side with your right foot.

4-Brush the floor with your left foot alongside your right foot.

1-Step out to the left side with your left foot.

2-Step behind your left foot with your right foot.

3-Step out to the left side with your left foot.

4-Stomp with your right foot beside your left foot.

        REPEAT

Music for the Cowboy Stomp
    (Honky–Tonk Stomp) Line Dance
-   *Eighteen Wheels and a Dozen Roses*.....Kathy Mattea.
-   *Fishin' in the Dark*.....The Nitty Gritty Dirt Band..

The Four Corners Line Dance

1,2-Move your right foot out to the right side and return it to normal stance.

3,4-Move your right foot out to the right side and return it to normal stance.

1,2-Move your left foot back and return it to normal stance.

3,4-Move your left foot out to the left side and return it to normal stance.

1,2-Pigeon toe.

3-Move your right leg forward and tap your heel to the floor.

4-Move your right leg to cross over in front of your left leg.

1-Move your right leg forward and tap your heel to the floor.

2-Bring your right leg back into your normal stance.

3-Move your left leg forward and tap your heel to the floor.

4-Move your left leg to cross over in front of your right leg.

1-Move your left leg forward and tap your heel to the floor.

2-Bring your left leg back, touching only your toes to the floor.

3-Step forward with your left foot.

4-Kick forward with your right foot.

1-Step back with your right foot.

2-Step back with your left foot and touch your toes to the floor.

3-Step forward with your left foot, do a quarter-turn to your left.

4-Hitch up with your right knee bent.

1-Step down and to the right with your right foot.

2-Step with your left foot behind your right foot.

3-Step out to the right with your right foot.

4-Brush the floor with your left foot alongside your right foot.

1-Step out to the left with your left foot.

2-Step with your right foot behind your left foot.

3-Step out to the left with your left foot.

4-Stomp your right foot beside your left foot.

REPEAT

Music for the Four Corners Line Dance

□   *Betty's Been Bad*.....Sawyer Brown.

□   *Guitars and Cadillacs*.....Dwight Yoakum.

The Lazy Slide Line Dance

1-Move your right foot forward and touch your heel to the floor.

2-Move your right foot to cross over in front of your left foot.

3-Move your right foot back to forward position and touch your heel to the floor.

4-Move your right foot back to normal stance.

1-Move your left foot forward and touch your heel to the floor.

2-Move your left foot to cross over in front of your right foot.

3-Move your left foot back to forward position and touch your heel to the floor.

4-Move your left foot back to normal stance.

1-Step out to the right with your right foot.

2-Slide your left foot to your right foot.

3-Step out to the right with your right foot.

4-Slide your left foot to your right foot.

1-Step to the left side with your left foot.

2-Slide your right foot to your left foot.

3-Step out to the left side with your left foot.

4-Slide your right foot to your left foot.

1-Step out to the right with your right foot.

2-Slide your left foot to your right foot.

3-Step out to the left with your left foot.

4-Slide your right foot to your left foot.

1,2-With a slight bend in your knees, do a quarter-turn to your left, pivoting on the balls of your feet. (Also known as the "corkscrew.")

3,4-Kick in a forward and downward motion with your right foot, twice.

1-Step back with your right foot.

2-Step back with your left foot.

3-Step back with your right foot.

4-Step back with your left foot.

1-Step forward with your right foot.

2-Hitch up with bent left knee.

3-Step down with your left foot.

4-Stomp your right foot alongside your left foot.

1-Do a heel swish to the left.

2-Bring heels back to center (normal).

3-Do a heel swish to the right.

4-Bring heels back to center (normal).

REPEAT

Music for Lazy Slide Line Dance

☐ *If The Devil Danced In Empty Pockets*.....Joe Diffie.

☐ *Backroads*.....Ricky Van Shelton.

The Freeze Line Dance

1-Step out to the right with your right foot.

2-Step behind your right foot with your left foot.

3-Step out to the right with your right foot.

4-Hitch up with your left knee bent.

1-Step out to the left side with your left foot.

2-Step behind your left foot with your right foot.

3-Step out to the left with your left foot.

4-Hitch up with your right knee bent.

1-Step backwards with your right foot.

2-Step backwards with your left foot.

3-Step backwards with your right foot.

4-Hitch up with your left knee bent.

1-Bring your left foot down in forward position and rock forward.

2-Rock back on your right foot.

3-Rock on your left foot forward doing quarter-turn to your left.

4-Brush the floor with your right leg.

REPEAT.

Music for the Freeze Line Dance

☐ *Better Man*.....Clint Black.

☐ *All is Fair in Love and War*.....Ronnie Milsap.

The Tush Push Line Dance

Option 1:

1,2,3,4-Tap your right heel to the floor from normal stance 4 times.

1,2,3,4-Tap your left heel to the floor from normal stance 4 times.

1-Do a heel swish to the left.

2-Do a heel swish to the right.

3,4-Do a heel swish to the left (clap hands).

Or ... Option 2:

1,2-Move your right heel forward, tap it to the floor and return.

3,4-Move your right heel forward and tap it to the floor twice.
Hop and switch your weight on your right foot.

1,2-Move your left heel forward, tap it to the floor and return.

3,4-Move your left heel forward and tap it to the floor twice.

1,2-Do a hip bump to the right twice.

3,4-Do a hip bump to the left twice.

1,2,3,4-Rotate hips in gyrating motion clockwise to a count of 4.

1,2,3-Do shuffle steps forward right, left, right.

4-Step forward on your left foot and rock forward on it.

1,2,3-Do shuffle steps backward left, right, left.

4-Rock back on your right foot.

1,2,3-Do shuffle steps forward right, left, right.

4-Step forward with your left foot and do a half-turn to the right, pivoting on the balls of your feet.

1,2,3-Do shuffle steps forward left, right, left.

4-Step forward with your right foot and do a half-turn to the left, pivoting on the balls of your feet.

1-Step forward with your right foot.

2-Do a quarter directional turn to your left on the balls of your feet.

3,4-Stomp your right foot alongside your left foot and clap hands.
REPEAT

Music for Tush Push Line Dance

☐ *Redneck Girl*.....Bellamy Brothers.

☐ *I Feel Lucky*.....Mary Chapin Carpenter.

The Texas Slide Line Dance

1-Step out to your right side with your right foot.

2-Step behind your right foot with your left foot.

3-Step out to your right side with your right foot.

4-Kick with a brushing motion towards your right side with your left foot.

1-Step out to your left side with your left foot.

2-Step behind your left foot with your right foot.

3-Step out to your left side with your left foot.

4-Kick with a brushing motion towards your left side with your right foot.

1-Step back with your right foot.

2-Step back with your left foot.

3-Step back with your right foot.

4-Bring your left knee up (halfway to hitch position).

1-Step down on your left foot; while doing so, squat downward and slightly forward with your body weight mostly on your left foot.

2-Tap the toes of your right foot behind and to the outside of your left foot.

3-Step down on your right foot.

4-Bring your left knee up in hitch position.

1-Step down on your left foot, preparing for a quarter-directional turn to your left.

2-Bring your right knee up in hitch position, completing the quarter-turn.

REPEAT

Music for Texas Slide Line Dance

☐   *Mirror, Mirror*.....Diamond Rio.

☐   *Better Man*.....Clint Black.

L.A. Walk Line Dance

1,2-Move your right foot out to the right and return it to normal stance.

3,4-Move your right foot out to the right and return it to normal stance.

1,2-Move your left foot out to the left and return it to normal stance.

3,4-Move your left foot out to the left and return it to normal stance.

1,2-Move your right leg forward and tap the heel of your right foot to the floor, twice.

3,4-Move your right leg backward and tap the toes of your right foot to the floor, twice.

1-Move your right leg forward and tap the heel of your right foot to the floor, once.

2-Move your right leg backward and tap the toes of your right foot to the floor, once.

3,4-Step forward with your right foot and pivot half-turn to your left.

1,2-Step forward with your right foot and pivot half-turn to your left.

3-Move your right leg forward and tap the heel of your right foot to the floor, once.

4-Move your right leg backward and tap the toes of your right foot to the floor, once.

1-Move your right foot a quarter-turn to the right.

2-Kick your left foot out to your left side, not touching the floor.

3-Step over in front of your right foot with your left foot.

4-Kick your right foot out to your right side, not touching the floor.

5-Step over in front of your left foot with your right foot.

6-Step back with your left foot.

7-Step back with your right foot.

8-Bring your left foot together with your right foot by stomping with your left foot, once.

REPEAT

Music for L.A. Walk Line Dance

☐   *All is Fair in Love and War*.....Ronnie Milsap.

☐   *Ain't Nothing Wrong with the Radio*.....Aaron Tippin.

The Electric Slide Line Dance

1-Step out to the right with your right foot.

&-Slide your left foot to your right foot.

2-Step out to the right with your right foot.

&-Slide your left foot to your right foot.

3-Step out to the right with your right foot.

4-Brush the floor with your left foot beside your right foot.

1-Step out to the left with your left foot.

&-Slide your right foot to your left foot.

2-Step out to the left with your left foot.

&-Slide your right foot to your left foot.

3-Step out to the left with your left foot.

4-Brush the floor with your right foot beside your left foot.

1-Step back with your right foot.

2-Step back with your left foot.

3-Step back with your right foot.

4-Move your left leg forward and tap your heel to the floor.

1-Rock forward on your left foot.

2-Tap the toes of your right foot to the floor (with your right leg back).

3-Rock back on your right foot.

4-Tap your left heel to the floor in front of you.

1-Rock forward on your left foot doing a quarter-turn to your left.

2-Brush your right foot alongside your left foot.

REPEAT

NOTE: *The step/slide sequences are done at a very quick pace, almost like shuffling from side to side.*

Music for the Electric Slide Line Dance

☐   *She's in Love with the Boy*.....Trisha Yearwood.

☐   *Bible Belt*.....Travis Tritt.

The California Cowboy Boogie
Line Dance

1- Step out to the right side with your right foot.

2- Step behind your right foot with your left foot.

3- Step out to the right side with your right foot.

4- Scuff the floor with the heel of your boot with your left foot alongside your right foot.

1- Step out to the left side with your left foot.

2- Step behind your left foot with your right foot.

3- Step out to the left side with your left foot.

4- Scuff the floor with the heel of your boot with your right foot alongside your left foot.

1-Step down in place with your right foot.

2-Scuff your left foot alongside your right foot.

3-Step down in place with your left foot.

4-Scuff your right foot in forward direction against your left foot.

1-Step back with your right foot.

2-Step back with your left foot.

3-Step with your right foot, and in the same movement do a quarter-turn to the right, pivoting on your right foot.

4-Brush your left foot alongside your right foot, and in the same motion step out to the left side with your left foot.

1,2-Do a hip bump to the left for 2 counts.

3,4-Do a hip bump to the right for 2 counts.

1-Do a hip wiggle to the left.

2-Do a hip wiggle to the center (with your butt pressed to the back).

3-Do a hip wiggle to the right.

4-Do half-turn to the left, pivoting on your left foot, and brush your right foot alongside your left foot.

REPEAT

Music for the California Boogie Line Dance

☐ *Next to You, Next to Me*.....Shenandoah.

☐ *Past the Point of Rescue*.....Hal Ketchum.

The Cowboy Boogie Line Dance

1-Step out to the right side with your right foot.

2-Step behind your right foot with your left foot.

3-Step out to the right side with your right foot.

4-Hitch up with your left knee bent.

1-Step down to the left with your left foot.

2-Step behind your left foot with your right foot.

3-Step out to the left side with your left foot.

4-Hitch up with your right knee bent.

1-Step down and forward with your right foot.

2-Scuff forward with your left foot alongside your right foot.

3-Step down on your left foot.

4-Scuff forward with your right foot.

1-Step back with your right foot.

2-Step back with your left foot.

3,4-Step back with your right foot and press your hips toward your right.

1,2-Do a hip shake to the left, twice.

3,4-Do a hip shake to the right, twice.

1-Rock forward with your weight on your left foot.

2-Rock back with your weight on your right foot.

3-Rock forward on your left foot while moving into a quarter-turn to your left.

4-Brush the floor with your right foot alongside your left foot.
REPEAT.

Music for the Cowboy Boogie Line Dance

☐ *Old Flames Have New Names*.....Mark Chesnutt.

☐ *Mirror, Mirror*.....Diamond Rio.

The Achy Breaky Line Dance

The best way to learn the Achy Breaky is to break it down in four segments of eight counts.

Example of count:

1-2-3, hold 4-5-6-7, hold 8.

1-2-3-(half-turn to your left)=4,-5-6-(hitch doing quarter-turn to your left)=7-8.

(Step back)=1-2-3 (stomp)=4,-5-6-7-hold 8.

Step-press-step-press-5-6-7-(stomp)=8.

Yes, it does sound complicated. This is one of the more difficult line dances to learn, but once you get it, you wonder how could this have taken so long to learn as it's easy. Note that with the song you need to count or lead yourself into the dance on a specific beat, so that your last step (which is a stomp) will end at the same ending beat as the song.

The first sequence of eight counts:

1-Step out to your right side with your right foot.

2-Step behind your right foot with your left foot.

3-Step out to your right side with your right foot.

4- Hold this position for (1) count; weight should be on the right foot with hips pressed to the right.

5-Swing your hips to the left.

6-Swing your hips to the right.

7-Swing your hips to the left.

8-Hold this position for 1 count; weight should be on your left foot with your hips pressed to the left.

The second sequence of eight counts:

1-Step with your right foot back, touching only your toes to the floor.

2-Bring your right foot out to your right side only touching your toes to the floor.

3-Do quarter-turn to your left by pivoting on your left foot extending your right foot out to your right side after completion of the quarter-turn.

4-Do half-turn (Face opposite direction you are after [3] count) bringing your right foot down in back position (Resting in the balls of your right foot).

5-Step back with your left foot.

6-Step back with your right foot.

7-Hitch upward with your left knee bent and do quarter-turn to your left.

8-Bring your left foot down alongside your right foot.

The third sequence of eight counts:

1-Step back with your right foot.

2-Step back with your left foot.

3-Step back with your right foot.

4-Bring your left foot alongside your right foot with a stomp.

5-Step out to your left side and swing your hips to the left.

6-Swing your hips to the right.

7-Swing your hips to the left.

8-(Hold) this position for (1) count; weight should be on the left foot with your hips pressed to the left.

The fourth sequence of eight counts:

1-Step turning your right foot quarter-turn to your right.

2-Step out to the left side with your left foot touching only the ball of your foot to the floor as if you were squishing a bug.

3-Bring your left foot back to the starting position by doing quarter-turn to your left and in the same motion after doing quarter-turn.

4-Do another quarter-turn to the right pressing out with the right foot like you're squishing another bug with the ball of your foot.

5-Raise your right foot off the floor approx. 6" and step out to the right.

6-Step behind your right foot with your left foot.

7-Step out to your right side with your right foot.

8-Stomp your left foot alongside your right foot.

REPEAT ALL FOUR SEQUENCES.

Music for the Achy Breaky Line Dance:

☐ *Achy Breaky Heart*.....Billy Ray Cyrus.

The Alley Cat Line Dance

1-Twist to the left with a heel swish and return to normal stance.

2-Twist to the left with a heel swish and return to normal stance.

3-Move your right leg forward and tap your heel to the floor and return.

4-Move your right leg forward and tap your heel to the floor and return.

1-Twist to the left with a heel swish and return to normal stance.

2-Twist to the left with a heel swish and return to normal stance.

3-Move your left leg forward and tap your heel to the floor and return.

4-Move your left leg forward and tap your heel to the floor and return.

1-Step forward with your left foot then slide your right foot to your left foot.

2-Step forward with your left foot then slide your right foot to your left foot.

3-Step forward with your left foot then slide your right foot to your left foot.

4-Step forward with your left foot then slide your right foot to your left foot.

1-Step back at a 45° angle with your right foot then slide your left foot to your R-foot.

2-Step back at a 45° angle with your left foot then slide your right foot to your L-foot.

3-Step back at a 45° angle with your right foot then slide your left foot to your R-foot.

4-Step back at a 45° angle with your left foot then slide your right foot to your L-foot.

1-Step out to your right side with your right foot.

2-Slowly slide your left foot to your right foot with a butt wiggle.

3-Step out to your right side with your right foot.

4-Slowly slide your left foot to your right foot with a butt wiggle.

1-Step out to your left side with your left foot.

2-Slowly slide your right foot to your left foot with a butt wiggle.

3-Step out to your left side with your left foot.

4-Slowly slide your right foot to your left foot with a butt wiggle.
   Kick, Ball-Change (kicking with right foot).
   Kick, Ball-Change (kicking with right foot).

1-Step forward with your right foot.

2-Bring your left foot alongside of your right foot.

3-Move your left foot out to the left side and touch the ball of your foot to the floor.

4-Bring your left foot back to normal stance.

1-Step out to the left side with your left foot.

2-Step behind your left foot with your right foot.

3-Step out to the left side turning your left foot quarter-turn to the left.

4-Brush the floor with your right boot in a forward direction.

1-Step back with your right foot.

2-Step back with your left foot.

3-Step back with your right foot.

4-Stomp your left foot alongside your right foot.

Music for Alley Cat Line Dance
☐   *Overnight Male*.....George Strait.
☐   *She Lays It All on The Line*.....George Strait.

The Slappin' Leather Line Dance (Version 1)

1,2-Move your right foot forward and tap your heel to the floor and return to normal stance.

3,4-Move your left foot forward and tap your heel to the floor and return.

1,2-Move your right foot forward and tap your heel to the floor and return.

3,4-Move your left foot forward and tap your heel to the floor and return.

1,2-Move your right foot forward and tap your heel to the floor, twice.

3,4-Move your right foot back and tap your toes to the floor, twice.

1-Move your right forward and tap your heel to the floor, once.

2-Move your right foot out to your right side and touch the ball of your foot to the floor.

3-Bring your right foot up behind your left knee and slap your right heel with your left hand.

4-Bring your right foot down and brush the floor with your right foot while doing a quarter-turn to your left... and in the same fluid motion.

5-Bring your right foot up in front of your left knee and slap your right heel with your left hand.

6-Swing your right foot out to the right (not touching the floor) and slap your right heel with your right hand.

1-Bring your right foot down, stepping out to the right side.

2-Step behind your right foot with your left foot.

3-Step out to the right side with your right foot.

4-Brush the floor with your left foot alongside your right foot.

1-Step to the left side with your left foot.

2-Step behind your left foot with your right foot.

3-Step to the left side with your left foot.

4-Brush forward with your right foot alongside your left foot.

1-Step back with your right foot.

2-Step back with your left foot.

3-Step back with your right foot.

4-Hitch up and forward with your left knee bent.

1,2-Step down on your left foot and slide your right foot to your left foot.

3,4-Step forward with your left foot and slide your right foot to your left foot.

1-Swish your heels to the left.

2-Return to normal stance.

3-Swish your heels to the right.

4-Return to normal stance.

REPEAT

Music for Slappin' Leather Line Dance

☐ *Bible Belt*.....Travis Tritt.

☐ *Get Rhythm*.....Martin DelRay.

☐ *Bang Bang*.....Kelly Willis.

☐ *Shakin'*.....Sawyer Brown.

Slappin' Leather (Version 2)

1,2-Move your right foot forward and tap your heel to the floor and return to normal stance.

3,4-Move your left foot forward and tap your heel to the floor and return.

1,2-Move your right foot forward and tap your heel to the floor and return.

3,4-Move your left foot forward and tap your heel to the floor and return.

1,2-Move your right foot forward and tap your heel to the floor, twice.

3,4-Move your right back and tap your toes to the floor, twice.

1-Bring your right foot up in front of your left knee and slap your right heel with your left hand.

2-Swing your right foot out to the right (not touching the floor) and slap your right heel with your right hand.

3-Swing your right foot behind your left knee and slap your right heel with your left hand.

4-Swing your right foot out to the right and slap your right heel with your right hand (with quarter-turn left).

5-Bring your right foot up in front of your left knee and slap your right heel with your left hand.

6-Swing your right foot out to the right, not touching the floor, and slap your right heel with your right hand.

1-Bring your right foot down, stepping out to the right side.

2-Step behind your right foot with your left foot.

3-Step out to the right side with your right foot.

4-Brush the floor with your left foot along side your right foot.

1-Step to the left side with your left foot.

2-Step behind your left foot with your right foot.

3-Step to the left side with your left foot.

4-Brush forward with your right foot alongside your left foot.

1-Step back with your right foot.

2-Step back with your left foot.

3-Step back with your right foot.

4-Hitch up and forward with your left knee.

1,2-Step forward with your left foot and slide your right foot to your left foot.

3,4-Step forward with your left foot and slide your right foot to your left foot.

1-Swish your heels to the left.

2-Return to normal stance.

3-Swish your heels to the right.

4-Return to normal stance.

REPEAT

Slappin' Leather (Version 3)

(10 count)

1,2-Move your right foot forward and tap your heel to the floor and return.

3,4-Move your left foot forward and tap your heel to the floor and return.

1,2-Move your right foot forward and tap your heel to the floor and return.

3,4-Move your left foot forward and tap your heel to the floor and return.

1-Move your right foot forward slightly and touch the floor with your heel.

2-Raise your right leg swinging your right foot out to the right side and slap your right heel with your right hand.

3-Straighten your right leg and touch the floor with your right heel.

4-Bring your right leg up in front of your left knee and slap your right heel with your left hand.

5-Straighten your right leg and touch the floor with your right heel.

6-Raise your right leg swinging your right foot out to the right side and slap your right heel with your right hand.

7-Without touching the floor, swing your right foot behind your left knee and slap your right foot with your right hand.

8-Swing your right foot out to the right and slap your right heel with your right hand, letting your momentum carry you through a quarter-turn to your left, pivoting on left foot.

9-Swing your right foot in front of your left knee and slap your right heel with your left hand.

10-Swing your right foot out to the right and slap your right heel with your right hand.

1-Step down and to your right with your right foot.

2-Step behind your right foot with your left foot.

3-Step out to the right with your right foot.

4-Brush the floor with your left foot alongside your right foot.

1-Step out to the left side with your left foot.

2-Step behind your left foot with your right foot.

3-Step to the left side with your left foot.

4-Brush forward with your right foot alongside your left foot.

1-Step back with your right foot.

2-Step back with your left foot.

3-Step back with your right foot.

4-Hitch up and forward with your left knee.

1,2-Step down on your left foot and slide your right foot to your left foot.

3,4-Step forward with your left foot and slide your right foot to your left foot.

1-Swish your heels to the left.

2-Return heels to the center.

3-Swish your heels to the right.

4-Return heels to center.

REPEAT

The Texas Corners Line Dance

1,2-Pigeon toe.

2,3-Pigeon toe.

1,2-Move your left leg forward and tap your heel to the floor and return.

3,4-Move your left leg forward and tap your heel to the floor and return.

1,2-Move your right leg forward and tap your heel to the floor and return.

3,4-Move your right leg forward and tap your heel to the floor and return.

1,2-Step forward with your left foot and kick with your right foot.

3-Step back with your right foot.

4-Move your left leg back and touch your toes to the floor.

1,2-Step forward with your left foot and kick with your right foot.

3-Step back with your right foot.

4-Move your left leg back and touch your toes to the floor.

1-Step forward with your left foot doing quarter-turn to your left.

2-Hitch up with your right knee.

3-Step to the right side with your right foot.

4-Step behind your right foot with your left foot.

1-Step to the right side with your right foot.

2-Stomp your left foot alongside your right foot.

REPEAT

Music for Texas Corners Line Dance
☐ *I'll Start With You*.....Paulette Carlson.
☐ *Killin' Time*.....Clint Black.

The Texas Twist Line Dance

1,2-Do a heel swish to the right and return to normal stance.

3,4-Do a heel swish to the right and return to normal stance.

1,2-Do a heel swish to the right and return to normal stance.

3,4-Do a heel swish to the right and return to normal stance.

1-Move your right leg forward and touch your heel to the floor.

2-Bring your right foot back alongside your left foot.

3-Step with your right foot out to your right side.

4-Do a quarter-turn pivot to your left.

1-Move your right foot out to your right side and touch your toes to the floor.

2-Bring your right knee up towards your left thigh.

3-Move your right foot out to your right side and touch your toes to the floor.

4-Bring your right knee up towards your left thigh.

1-Step out to the right side with your right foot.

2-Step behind your right foot with your left foot.

3-Step out to the right side with your right foot.

4-Stomp your left foot down alongside your right foot.

1-Move your left foot out to your left side and touch your toes to the floor.

2-Bring your left knee up towards your right thigh.

3-Move your left foot out to your left side and touch your toes to the floor.

4-Bring your left knee up towards your right thigh.

1-Step out to your left side with your left foot.

2-Step behind your left foot with your right foot.

3-Step out to your left side with your left foot.

4-Stomp your right foot down alongside your left foot.

REPEAT

Music for Texas Twist Line Dance

☐ *Will I Do*.....Prairie Oyster.

☐ *Wild Horses*.....Garth Brooks.

The Sluefoot Stomp Line Dance

1,2-Pigeon toe.

3-Move your right leg forward and touch your heel to the floor.

4-Bring your right foot back alongside your left foot.

1-Step out to the right side with your right foot.

2-Step behind your right foot with your left foot.

3-Step out to the right side with your right foot.

4-Stomp your left foot down alongside your right foot.

1,2-Pigeon toe.

3-Move your left leg forward and touch your heel to the floor.

4-Bring your left foot back alongside your right foot.

1-Step out to the left side with your left foot.

2-Step behind your left foot with your right foot.

3-Step out to the left side with your left foot.

4-Stomp your right foot down alongside your left foot.

1,2-With your right foot (only), do a heel swish to the right and return.

3,4-With your left foot (only), do a heel swish to the left and return.

1,2-Pigeon toe.

3,4-Pigeon toe.

1-Step forward with your right foot.

2-Step forward with your left foot.

3-Step forward with your right foot.

4-Scuffing the floor with your left heel in forward motion, bring your left knee up.

1-Step down and forward with your left foot.

2-Step forward with your right foot.

3-Step forward with your left foot preparing for quarter-directional turn to the left by pointing your toes to the left.

4-Stomp the floor with your right foot alongside your left foot.
REPEAT

Music for Sluefoot Stomp Line Dance
- ☐ *Guitars & Cadillacs*.....Dwight Yoakum.
- ☐ *Don't Rock The Jukebox*.....Alan Jackson.

The Electric Boogie Line Dance
(The T.C. Slide)

1-Step out to your right side with your right foot.

2-Step behind your right foot with your left foot.

3-Step out to your right side with your right foot.

4-Brush forward with your left foot.

1-Step out to your left side with your left foot.

2-Step behind your left foot with your right foot.

3-Step out to your left side with your left foot.

4-Brush forward with your right foot.

1-Step back with your right foot.

2-Step back with your left foot.

3-Step back with your right foot.

4-Bring your left foot beside your right foot.

1-Jump up with your feet landing apart.

2-Jump up with your feet landing together.

3-Bring your left foot out and step down with it crossed over in front of your right foot.

4-Bring your right foot around and step down crossed over in front of your left foot.

1,2-Step at a 45° angle to your left with your left foot, then slowly drag your right foot to your left foot.

3,4-Step at a 45° angle to your right with your right foot, then slowly drag your left foot to your right foot.

1,2-Do a hip bump forward and out with your left hip, twice.

3,4-Do a hip bump back and out with your right hip, twice.

1-Bump your left hip forward.

2-Bump your right hip back.

3,4-Bump your left hip forward and rotating so when you brush with your right foot you'll be completing a quarter-turn to your left.

REPEAT

Music for Electric Boogie Line Dance

☐ *Take A Little Trip*.....Alabama.

☐ *Uptown, Downtown*.....Mark Chesnutt.

The Ski-Bumpus Line Dance

The "Kick, Ball-Change": *First, kick with your right foot; now, stepping down on the ball of your right foot, quickly step down in place, distributing your weight to your left foot.*

1,2-Move your right foot out to the right side and touch the ball of your foot to the floor and return.

3,4-Move your left foot out to the left side and touch the ball of your foot to the floor and return.

1,2-Move your right foot out to the right side and touch the ball of your foot to the floor and return.

3,4-Move your left foot out to the left side and touch the ball of your foot to the floor and return.

1&2-Kick forward with your right foot, following up with a ball, chain.

3&4-Kick forward with your right foot, following up with a ball, chain.

1,2-Step forward with your right foot and do a half-turn (military turn) pivoting to the left.

1&2-Kick forward with your right foot, following up with a ball, chain.

3&4-Kick forward with your right foot, following up with a ball, chain.

1,2-Step forward with your right foot and do a half-turn to the left.

1&2-Shuffle steps: right, left, right.

3&4-Shuffle steps: left, right, left.

1,2-Step forward with your right foot and do a half-turn to the left.

1&2-Shuffle steps: right, left, right.

3&4-Shuffle steps: left, right, left.

1,2-Step forward with your right foot and do a half-turn to the left.

1,2,3,4-(Jazz Box)=Stepping forward set your right foot down crossed over in front of your left foot Step back with your left foot Step back with your right foot. Stomp with your left foot in place alongside your right foot.

1,2,3,4-(Jazz Box)=Stepping forward set your right foot down crossed over in front of your left foot Step back with your left foot Step back with your right foot Stomp with your left foot in place alongside your right foot.
REPEAT

Music for Ski-Bumpus Line Dance
- ☐ *Brand New Man*.....Brooks & Dunn.
- ☐ *Some Folks Like To Steal*.....Kentucky Head Hunters.

The Flying Eight Line Dance

1-Step out to your left side with your left foot.
2-Step behind your left foot with your right foot.
3-Step out to your left side with your left foot.
4-Hitch up with your right knee bent.
1-Step out to your right side with your right foot.
2-Step behind your right foot with your left foot.
3-Step out to your right side with your right foot.
4-Hitch up with your left knee bent doing quarter-turn to your right.
1-Step out to your left side with your left foot.
2-Step behind your left foot with your right foot.
3-Step out to your left side with your left foot.
4-Hitch up with your right knee bent and do a three-quarter-turn to your left.
1-Rock forward on your right foot.
2-Rock back on your left foot.
3-Rock forward on your right foot.
4-Kick forward with your left foot.
1-Step forward with your left foot.
2-Kick forward with your right foot.
3-Step forward with your right foot.
4-Kick forward with your left foot.
REPEAT

Music for Flying Eight Line Dance
- ☐ *I Feel Lucky*.....Mary Chapin Carpenter.
- ☐ *Little Sister*.....Dwight Yoakum.

The Peter Push Line Dance

1-With your right foot(Scrape)pull your foot back like your wiping it off on the floor & return.

2-Scrape with your left foot and return.

3-Scrape with your right foot and return.

4-Scrape with your left foot and return.

1&2-Shuffle step forward: right, left, right.

3&4-Shuffle step forward: left, right, left.

1,2-Kick your right foot forward, twice (not touching the floor between kicks).

3,4-Jump back with your feet landing together and draw your pistols.

1,2,3,4-Now leaving your guns up in drawn position walk forward bowlegged: right, left, right, left.

1,2-Do a hip bump, twice while doing a quarter-turn to your right.

1-Step out to your right side with your right foot.

2-Step behind your right foot with your left foot.

3-Step out to your right side with your right foot.

4-Brush in forward motion with your left foot.

1-Step out to your left side with your left foot.

2-Step behind your left foot with your right foot.

3-Step out to your left side with your left foot.

4-Spin on your left foot doing a half-turn to the left with your right foot in the air.

1-Step down and stomp with your right foot.

2-Stomp your left foot beside your right foot.

3-Stomp in place with your right foot and holster your right gun.

4-Stomp in place with your left foot and holster your left gun.

REPEAT

Music for Peter Push Line Dance

☐ *Loves Got A Hold On You*.....Alan Jackson.

☐ *Long White Cadillac*.....Dwight Yoakum.

The Locomotion Line Dance

1,2-Step out to your right side, slide your left foot beside your right foot.

3,4-Step out to your left side, slide your right foot beside your left foot.

1,2-Step out to your right side, slide your left foot beside your right foot.

3,4-Step out to your left side, slide your right foot beside your left foot.

1,2-Step at a 45° angle to your right then bring your left foot to your right foot.

3,4-Step at a 45° angle to your right then bring your left foot to your right foot.

1,2-Step at a 45° angle to your left then bring your right foot to your left foot.

3,4-Step at a 45° angle to your left then bring your right foot to your left foot.

1-Step forward with your right foot.

2-Step forward with your left foot.

3-Step forward with your right foot.

4-Kick forward with your left foot.

1-Step back with your left foot.

2-Step back with your right foot.

3-Step back with your left foot.

4-Bring your right foot together alongside your left foot.

1-Jump forward (feet together).

2-Jump backward.

3-Jump forward.

4-Jump doing a quarter-turn to the right and landing feet together.

REPEAT

Music for Locomotion Line Dance
☐ *Long White Cadillac*.....Dwight Yoakum.
☐ *Honky Tonk Man*.....Dwight Yoakum.

Hooked–On–Country Line Dance

1&2-Start with your right leg and do shuffle steps back, ... right, left, right.

3&4-Move your left leg and do shuffle steps back ... left, right, left.

1-Step forward with your right foot.

2-Step forward with your left foot.

3-Step forward with your right foot.

4-Kick forward with your left foot.

1-Step back with your left foot.

2-Step back with your right foot.

3-Step back with your left foot.

&4-(Kick, Ball-Change)=Step down on your right foot, then quickly shift your weight on your left foot.

1-Step out to your right side with your right foot.

2-Step behind your right foot with your left foot.

3-Step out to your right side with your right foot.

4-Kick out in front at a 45° angle with your left foot toward your right.

1-Step down and out to your left with your left foot.

2-Step behind your left foot with your right foot.

3-Step out to your left with your left foot.

4-Kick out in front at a 45° angle with your right foot towards your left.

1-Stepping down, bring your right foot beside your left foot.

2-Kick forward with your left foot.

3-Stepping down, bring your left foot beside your right foot.

4-Kick forward with your right foot.

1,2-Move your right leg back, and tap your toes to the floor twice.

3,4-Move your right leg forward, and tap your right heel to the floor twice.

1-Step forward on your right foot.

2-Do a quarter-turn, pivoting to your left.

3-Stomp your right foot beside your left foot.

4-Stomp your right foot beside your left foot.

REPEAT

Music for Hooked–On–Country Line Dance

☐ *Brand New Man.....Brooks & Dunn.*

☐ *Some Folks Like to Steal.....Kentucky Head Hunters.*

The Hitchhiker Line Dance

1,2-With your right hand, hitch-hike, (closed fist with thumb up), to the right, twice.

3,4-With your left hand, hitchhike to the left, twice.

1,2-With your right hand, (palms open and facing the front), wave in a circular motion, twice.

3,4-With your left hand wave in a circular motion, twice.

1,2-With both your arms bent at 90° and against your stomach, roll one over the other towards your right side, for two counts.

3,4-With the same motion: roll in the middle for two counts.

1,2-With the same motion: roll to the left for two counts.

3,4-With the same motion: roll in the middle for two counts.

1-Slap your left knee with your right hand.

2-Slap your right knee with your left hand.

3-Slap your right butt cheek with your right hand.

4-Slap your left butt cheek with your left hand.

1,2-With your right hand, make like you're drawing a pistol from it's holster, and shoot.

3,4-With your left hand, make like you're drawing a pistol from its holster, and shoot.

1,2-With guns up, jump up doing a quarter-turn to your right.

3,4-After landing, hold the position for one count, holster your guns, and clap your hands.
REPEAT

Music for the Hitchhiker Line Dance.

☐ *Some Folks Like to Steal*.....Kentucky Head Hunters.
☐ *San Antonio Stroll*.....Tanya Tucker.
☐ *Boogie Woogie Fiddle Blues*.....Charlie Daniels Band.

The Boot–Scootin' Boogie Line Dance

1,2,3,4-Twist to your left—toe, heel, toe, heel (known as zazzer step).

1,2,3,4-Twist to your right—heel, toe, heel, toe (zazzer step).

1,2-Move your right foot forward, and heel-strut (heel,toe).

3,4-Move your left foot forward, and heel-strut (heel,toe)

1,2-With your right foot, kick forward twice (not touching the floor between kicks).

3-Step back with your right foot.

4-Bring your left leg back and tap your toes to the floor.

1,2-Stepping forward with your left foot, and with your right knee bent in hitch position, scoot forward.

1&2-Stepping down on your right foot, do shuffle steps: right, left, right.

3&4-Shuffle steps: left, right, left.

1,2-Stepping forward with your right foot, do a half-turn pivot to your left.

1&2-Shuffle steps: right, left, right.

3&4-Shuffle steps: left, right, left.

1,2-Bringing your right knee up in hitch position, scoot forward twice.

1-Step out to your right side with your right foot.

2-Step behind your right foot with your left foot.

3-Step out to your right side with your right foot.

4-Tap the toes of your left foot to the floor directly in front of your right foot.

1,2-Move your left foot out to your left side, touching only your toes to the floor, clap & hold for 1 count.

1-Step out to your left side with your left foot.

2-Step behind your left foot with your right foot.

3-Step out to your left side with your left foot.

4-Tap the toes of your right foot to the floor directly in front of your left foot.

1,2-Move your right foot out to your right side touching toes (only) to the floor, clap & hold for 1 count.

1-Step a quarter-directional turn to the right with your right foot.

2-Slide your left foot crossed behind your right foot.

3-Stomp in place with your right foot.

4-Stomp in place with your left foot.

REPEAT

Music for Boot Scootin' Boogie Line Dance

☐ *Boot Scootin' Boogie*.....Brooks & Dunn.

The Twist Line Dance

1,2-Tap your right toe out to the right side and return.

3,4-Tap your right toe out to the right side and return.

1,2-Step out to the right side with your right foot then bring your left foot beside your right.

3,4-Step out to the right side with your right foot then bring your left foot beside your right.

1,2-Tap your left toe out to the left side and return.

3,4-Tap your left toe out to the left side and return.

1,2-Step out to the left side with your left foot then bring your right foot beside your left.

3,4-Step out to the left side with your left foot then bring your right foot beside your left.

1,2,3,4,5,6,7,8-Twist in place to an eight count.

1,2-Move your right leg forward and tap your heel to the floor, twice.

3,4-Move your right leg backward and tap your toes to the floor, twice.

1-Move your right leg forward and tap your heel to the floor.

2-Move your right leg backward and tap your toes to the floor.

3-Move your right leg into your normal stance.

4-Do a quarter-pivot turn to your left.

REPEAT

Music for Twist Line Dance

☐ *Bop*.....Dan Seals.

☐ *Don't Rock the Jukebox*.....Alan Jackson.

The Cowboy Strut Line Dance

1-Move your right leg forward and tap your heel to the floor.

2-Move your right foot to cross over in front of your left foot (only touching your toes to the floor).

3-Move your right leg forward and tap your heel to the floor.

4-Move your right foot out to your right side and touch your toes to the floor.

5-Move your right leg forward and tap your heel to the floor.

6-Return your right leg to normal stance.

1-Move your left leg forward and tap your heel to the floor.

2-Move your left foot to cross over in front of your right foot (only touching your toes to the floor).

3-Move your left leg forward and tap your heel to the floor.

4-Move your left foot out to your left side and touch your toes to the floor.

5-Move your left leg forward and tap your heel to the floor.

6-Move your left leg backward and tap your toes to the floor.

1-Step forward with your left foot.

2-Kick forward with your right foot.

3-Step back with your right foot.

4-Move your left leg backward and tap your toes to the floor.

1-Step out to your left side with your left foot.

2-Step behind your left foot with your right foot.

3-Step out to your left side with your left foot.

4-With your right foot, brush the floor while doing a half-turn to your left.

1,2,3,4-Strut forward (touch the heel then the toes to the floor as you strut): right, left, right, left.

1-Turn your right foot a quarter-turn to the right.

2-Step with your left foot so it's slightly back of your right foot, facing the same way.

3-Step in place with your right foot.

4-Step with your left foot so it's beside your right foot.

1,2,3,4-(JAZZ BOX)=Step with your right foot crossing over your left foot. Step slightly back with your left foot. Step slightly back with your right foot. Step, bringing your left foot beside your right foot.

REPEAT

Music for Cowboy Strut Line Dance
- ☐ *Men.....*Forester Sisters.
- ☐ *Workin' Man.....*Nitty Gritty Dirt Band.

Glossary of Country-Western Dancing Terminology

Brush — Sweep either foot along the floor in forward motion.

Fan — Standing with your feet together, toe-swish one of your feet either to the right or left, and return.

Grapevine Left — Step out to your left side with your left foot. Step behind your left foot with your right foot. Step out to your left side with your left foot.

Grapevine Right — Step out to your right side with your right foot. Step behind your right foot with your left foot. Step out to your right side with your right foot.

Heel Swish (Heel Swivel) — Standing with your feet together, swish your heels in same direction (with your weight on the balls of your feet), either right or left, and return to normal stance.

Hitch — Knee up at 90° — thigh parallel to the floor with lower part of leg hanging down.

Kick — Self-explaining. Just don't kick too high and hit someone.

Kick, Ball-Change — Kick in a forward motion with one foot, then step down on that foot, quickly shifting your weight to the other foot.

Military Turn — A half-turn either to the right or left, pivoting on the balls of your feet.

Pigeon Toe — Turn your toes inward, while you separate your heels outward, and return.

Scoot — A slide of the weighted foot, raising the other leg with a bent knee.

Scrape — Pull foot back against the floor as if you're using your steps to scrape mud off your boots.

Scuff — In forward motion, hit the floor with your boot heel as if to make a mark on the floor.

Shuffle Steps — For a full explanation, see the instructions for the Three-Step.

Toe Swish (Toe Swivel) — Standing with your feet together and weight on your heels, swish your toes in same direction, either to the right or left, and return to normal stance.

Index